Speaking and Learning the FASD Way

A Teacher's Journey into the World of Fetal Alcohol Spectrum Disorder

by

Carol McAndrew

RED LEAD PRESS
PITTSBURGH, PENNSYLVANIA 15222

ISBN-10: 0-8059-8277-9
ISBN-13: 978-0-8059-8277-0
Printed in the United States of America

First Printing

For information or to order additional books, please write:
Red Lead Press
701 Smithfield Street
Pittsburgh, Pennsylvania 15222
U.S.A.
1-800-834-1803
or visit our website and online catalogue at www.redleadbooks.com.

Working with Fetal Alcohol Spectrum students is challenging. The students I have encountered have taught me a great deal about FASD. It is an ongoing process, one I enjoy as I am learning new things and opening up to new possibilities.

I dedicate this book to Pat Richardson who has been a big inspiration and support to me throughout the process of writing.

Words to Educate By

"I have come to a frightening conclusion. I am the decisive element in the classroom. It is my personal approach that creates the climate. It is my daily mood that makes the weather.

As a teacher I possess tremendous power to make a child's life miserable or joyous. I can be a toll of torture or an instrument of inspiration. I can humiliate or humour, hurt or heal. In all situations it is my response that decides whether a crisis will be escalated or de-escalated, and a child humanized or dehumanized."

Dr. Haim Ginott

What FASD Young People Have to Say

"Having FASD means it is very hard to do things. Nothing is easy. I want to be treated with kindness and thoughtfulness-not like I am stupid."

"Be patient with me and encourage me. I learn slower."

"Employers want you to be perfect and they seem to want you to work fast."

"When I was younger, I would throw tantrums and hit people, steal and get involved with the wrong crowd."

From *Dear World: We Have Fetal Alcohol Syndrome* FASD Support Network (B.C.)

"We must move from viewing the individual as failing if he does not do well in a program to viewing the program as not providing what the individual needs in order to succeed." Dubovsky

Introduction

The truth is out. Fetal Alcohol Spectrum Disorder is real and affects many children and adults from all walks of life. It is time for all caregivers, teachers, para-professionals, support workers, law enforcement and medical personnel to gain an understanding of this invisible disabled population and create environments to help them become productive members of society. It is also time for society at large to advocate for healthy babies and support women in not drinking during pregnancy because FASD can be prevented.

Fetal Alcohol Syndrome is a result of the birth mother drinking during her pregnancy. The brain of the unborn child is affected causing irreparable neurological damage. Many birth mothers did not know that alcohol would hurt their unborn child. Some were addicts to alcohol. Regardless, most are fearful of admitting that they drank when they were pregnant. They carry a great deal of guilt for causing the defects in their child/children. Recently, through support groups such as The Fetal Alcohol Support Network in British Columbia birth moms are stepping forward to tell their stories. Their hope is to help prevent others from having FASD children. Having heard these life stories at many conferences as well as the sharing of young people with FASD I am compelled to write this book. No one exposed to these stories can be unmoved. Working with FASD youth has become my passion. I hope that what I share with you through the chapters to follow will give you a greater understanding of the difficulties this population of people face daily as well as seeing the gifts and talents within them.

No two people with FASD are alike but there are some similarities. These include slower processing speed, problems storing and retrieving information, gaps in learning, difficulty forming links, associations, understanding abstract concepts, difficulty generalizing, difficulty seeing the next steps, outcomes, disconnections-saying one thing but doing another, grasping pieces rather than concepts.

It is possible to identify specific educational strategies that help alcohol-affected children learn at school and in the home. Bathing the fetal brain in alcohol is like spilling a drink on a computer. Its circuits get scrambled in unpredictable ways. Much of the behaviour that parents and teachers find so aggravating is due to the problems the child's brain has in processing information. FASD children suffer from organic brain damage that makes it difficult for them to take in information, distinguish the signal from background noise in their environments, organize information in an integrated or sequential order and respond to the signal with the right routine.

Structure and consistency is key. Cutting down the amount of information a child has to deal with along with simple and concise directions helps the child cope. Visual cues and lists are invaluable as the child matures into adolescence and adulthood. As one FASD teenager told me, "There are too many words." It is important to keep verbal exchanges brief and to the point. FASD students need to have a mentor and advocate in the school setting, especially as they enter the secondary system. They need someone to pull them into participating in club and team activities and literally be their memory.

The following are areas that will be discussed and developed:

- Functions of Behaviour
- Receptive Language/Communication
- Environment/Structure
- Social Skills
- Job and Leisure Skills

FASD people require patience, love and firmness and a great deal of one-to-one teaching. The burden of the effects of FASD on the person, caregivers and teachers is great.

My challenge to you by the end of this book is to create your own FASD paradigm shift. Is the FASD student or adult truly a burden, or simply an incredible opportunity for you to use your knowledge and skills to help them find a way to survive in a world that has many barriers to success? How can we help FASD people become a credit rather than a debit to society?

The Pledge of the Teacher in the 21st Century

Although I think I 'm not good at coping,

The only thing I can't do is

NOTHING!

However,

I am allowed to

cry

whine

complain

be impatient

be frustrated

be bad tempered

think of quitting

but only if I

try my hardest

to find solutions

over-come obstacles

and do my best!

C. McAndrew

Chapter 1

Functional Behaviour Assessment -
Helping to Understand Behaviour

Many if not all FASD students are labelled early on as behaviour problems in school, at home and in the community. School files quickly grow in size as layers of behaviour assessments and plans are made. If only the presenting behaviours are looked at then the plans are doomed to failure. The negative behaviours continue and in most cases escalate. It is imperative that the underlying causes of the outward behaviours be analyzed. Only then can strategies be put in place to help the student with FASD be successful in a variety of situations.

A concept that is very helpful to use is behaviour mapping. In conjunction with the Langley District Training Team, district staff have come up with a model that is easy to use and offers a way to understand problem behaviours. This starts with completing a story about the student. (See figure 1) From there a hypothesis of what is the function of the behaviour can be developed. (See figure 2) From there an achievable behaviour plan can be developed. For example: from the boxes on setting events, triggering antecedents, problem behaviours, and negative reinforcers build a list of strategies that match the areas of discovered/possible need. If the setting event box suggest that one possible area of concern for the student is being overly tired, than a possible strategy might include working with the family on building bedtime routines. If the antecedent box suggests that the behaviour is more frequent after recess and lunch, a strategy might be to establish a check-in system for the student to help address any issues that might be arising from the free-time period. Remember to always build the plan from the student's strengths. What you hypothesize as the possible purpose of the behaviour needs to be also addressed by interim behaviours, for example, if the student is able to avoid work by engaging in the problem behaviour, then the interim behaviour needs to give the student a means to ask for a break, ask for help with work or be given options around the task.

The following strategy ideas may be useful in completing figure 3. Fill in the boxes with strategies to match the identified student need and choose a number of strategies that you wish to work on with the student- this is easily transferable to the student's Individual Educational Plan (IEP). If after several weeks the student's behaviour has not changed, you might want to try some of the other strategies you have developed from this plan and attempt them prior to re-assessing the behaviour map.

Some other factors to consider as you build this map- YOU ARE NOT ALONE! Who can help support you with this student? Can another teacher assist with the student taking a break in their room? Can another staff member assist with problem solving/class coverage so that you can problem solve with the student/others when difficulties arise? Can a Teacher Assistant (TA) or Child Care Worker (CCW) teach conflict resolution, social skills, anger management to the student? Can the Resource Teacher help with adapting/modifying curriculum or provide resources? Can a noon hour supervisor assist with monitoring and supervising on the playground? Can parents support with organizational skills, routines, nutrition? Can the student participate in the homework club? Can the principal or other key personnel assist with positive feedback to the student? Can community resources be accessed and put into place?

Contributing Factors Strategies: modifying and adapting curriculum as necessary, modifying or adapting the environment, physically separating the student from students with whom they have the most negative interactions, assessing academic skills, supporting bus times to school with monitors, supporting parents- hooking them up with community resources, providing food supplements at school, referring for counselling, community support and/or supporting with the medication program.

Precipitating Factors Strategies: clearly defining expectations, offering choices, increasing supervision/ monitoring, developing a check-in system, pairing with peers who are good role models, reducing the number of activities involving peers, reducing the number of changes in activities, breaking activity down into smaller steps, cueing to transitions, cueing to behaviour, using humour, redirection, clarification and or/reducing distractions.

Behaviour Teaching Strategies: teaching expectations, teaching students to break activities down into smaller parts, teaching students to take appropriate breaks and to ask for the breaks appropriately, teaching how to access help appropriately, teaching problem-solving/conflict resolution skills, anger management skills, friendship building skills, social skills, play skills/following the rules of games, self-monitoring strategies, positive self-talk, relaxation skills, deep breathing activities, homework skills and organizational skills.

Reinforcement Strategies: building relationships, follow-through, consistency, modelling, reward/reinforcing expectations, emphasizing connections between actions and words, rewarding appropriate behaviour/ and or celebrating progress and effort.

The plan that is built out of this behaviour map addresses the individual student by assessing alternate/replacement behaviour strategies. Individual, small group, and whole class/school planning can assist in addressing the desired behaviours on this map. Desired behaviours might include demonstrating respect, empathy and cooperation. (See figure 5)

I cannot emphasize enough the importance of doing a full functional behaviour assessment. Another tool I have found invaluable is to spend time before the start of a new school year with parents/care-givers to set up a mode of communication and dialogue. I ask them to complete a student profile for me which includes the student's strengths, likes, dislikes, what has worked in the past, what didn't work, what they perceive as the student's needs and any concerns they may have. (See figure6) This is so valuable in getting started in the right way to foster a successful year right from day one. It fosters proactiveness rather than reactiveness. Daily home-school communication is vital. I use a combination of a home communication book and e-mail or phone calls. E-mail is great because if the students "forget" their book I can still get the information to the home quickly. The student also sees that we are "talking".

The biggest difference in my success in working with challenging students has been my change of perspective in how I view challenging behaviours. I consciously tried over a period of time to catch my students being "good" Saying such things as "I appreciate you sharing your markers with Bob. That is being considerate." Students really responded to this and the feedback is telling them what they are doing right. That led my to go one step further. I started to monitor myself for phrasing my direction or redirection in a positive way. Rather than saying such things as "Don't hit" or "Don't put your feet on the desk" I would say "Keep you hands and feet to yourself" and "Please put your feet on the floor under your desk". It gives clear direction to the student when things are phrased in the positive. For FASD students this helps them make sense of the world and for both parties we are calmer and more relaxed. Be sure that when using praise that you clearly identify the behaviour not the student. For example, "Thank you for carrying the recycling bin, John. That was very helpful." Rather than, "Good boy, John, you are my best helper." If students do not appropriately follow the directions you give, use positive corrective feedback that does not put the

3

student down. For example, "I can't believe you hit Mary in the head with the recycling bin. You seem to care about no one but yourself!" Use, "John, stop. You need to walk around other students' desks with the recycling bin. Show me." Then have the student carry out the correct action.

After living through the teen years with 3 of my own children, I have come to realize the value of humour to diffuse many a tense situation. This is true with FASD students. Rather than getting myself worked into a frenzy complete with escalated blood pressure and a need to be reactive, making a joke or humourous redirection about a situation is a welcome diversion for all and in many cases a saving of face and a chance to regroup for the child.

Students with FASD are more likely to build positive self-concepts if they feel valued for who they are and will work more successfully. Success in school, in the home and in the community hinges on the consistent application of appropriate adaptations. It is important to note that however challenging a situation might be, the student is a person first, a person who happens to have FASD. Honouring the inner spirit- the essence of the student is so vital.

Many of my students have not recognized that they have FASD. They know something is different about them but they deny that they have the disorder. They will see it in others and often point out quite bluntly the other person's shortcomings. This is a teachable moment to be able to develop empathy for others but also to work with them to help them understand their diagnosis. Meeting and interacting with others with FASD at conferences and workshops is helpful. As a student said in a workshop for teachers and other professionals, "I have FASD but I am still a normal person. Please don't tease me. You shouldn't judge people before you know why they act the way they do."

No matter what the age of the individuals with FASD when I monitored their outbursts or meltdowns nearly all the time the cause was lack of understanding in what to do. Fear of new people and situations also fuelled heated outbursts and unkind words. Once I could define this through the use of the functional behaviour assessment I could set up strategies to help alleviate the anxiety. The storms were less frequent. As a student shared, "The emotional part of FASD can really get me into trouble. I get this bad attitude and it makes everyone around me miserable. Sometimes I get so frustrated I cry."

The functional behaviour assessment might seem onerous but it is truly worth the effort. It is a "road map" to give students sign posts and guides to help them become more effective in managing their behaviours. For each new day and each situation strategies and expectations must be reviewed, modelled and practiced. You can never practice enough!! Corrective actions need to be done immediately. Students quickly forget what they were in trouble for. Actions speak louder than words for this population.

Looking beyond the inappropriate behaviour is the key. FASD students are not good at expressing their feelings and thoughts well and behaviours at school or at home can be the result of an event that to us as adults may seem trivial but to the students it hurts deeply and they lash out. Repetition and reassurance is needed with each situation and expectations reviewed constantly throughout the day. Many FASD students come to my class with so much failure and rejection in the past and it takes time and patience to create a bond with them. I am their advocate no matter what. Awareness, acceptance and the willingness to understand a complex disorder, combined with an environment that "makes room" for differences is what makes the FASD students successful in school and in life.

A Lesson for the Teacher
By C. McAndrew

The way we see the world
Drawn from experiences good and bad
A need to rearrange the view
Continually searching to find new dimensions.

Gentle manipulation to rebuild perception
Unique, different-
A way to appreciate others
Stepping into their dimension
Looking through their eyes.

Gaining tolerance, patience and insight
Garnering a deeper understanding of what is important
Broadening mindsets and mustering resolve
Celebrations and tears
Being there no matter what.

Chapter 2

Receptive Language Development

FASD can be described as a problem of processing information-receiving information accurately, interpreting and remembering it correctly, and then acting on that information. Problems with central auditory processing (listening) encompass many aspects that impact the student's ability to follow directions and complete tasks.

Students with FASD are not able to keep up with the normal pace and complexity of the language of instruction and discussion, remember what has been said, and translate that into action. Visual cues and aides help with this. FASD students understand language messages in a concrete and literal way. They do not respond often to generalized statements or directions. For example, the teacher may say, "Get ready for PE." Or "Settle down." They do respond to more explicit instructions such as "Put on your gym shoes, now" or "lips together". Using their name helps them to focus on the speaker and know that the directions apply to them.

FASD students have trouble interpreting the intent of another speaker. Students with this type of language disability may be described as self-centred because they cannot take the listener's point of view. They will often go off on a completely different tangent as they respond to internal associations or experience that the speaker knows nothing about. They may just use pronouns to blurt out information in a discussion time with no referents or give so few details that the story they are trying to tell does not make sense. The words can be jumbled and speech very rapid and garbled. This sets up for conflicts. The student's anxiety increases and the event may end in an outburst. The student may be seen to be refusing to comply with a request but most often are unable to understand the request or task. What appears to be wilful disobedience actually is an inability to translate verbal directions into action.

To cover up inadequacies, FASD students may confabulate stories about events in the past or things that might happen. As an example, Billy tells me, "Guess what Ms Mc? Last night I played baseball. I hit lots of home runs and I struck out every batter. Then I hit a guy and broke his nose. Nobody could tag me out." In effect, Billy did play ball but was struck out each time and the other kids wanted to "hit" him because he couldn't follow the rules properly. Distinguishing between fact and fantasy can be hard for FASD people.

Here are some strategies I have found to be helpful in working with FASD language difficulties:

- Speak face-to face with the student and use the student's name.
- Keep the instructions short and concise.
- Stop at key points to check for comprehension
- Make sure the student knows what to do. They may be able to give you the instructions back but that doesn't mean they know what to do. Have them give you the instructions in their own words.
- Use visual cues and prompts along with verbal messages.
- Use lists, such as checklists for daily routines or work times.
- Slow down the tempo and wait for students to process. This takes a lot of practice on my part!!
- Be concrete and specific- non compliance may mean that the message was too ambiguous.
- Help the student feel comfortable asking for clarification
- Use repetitive teaching strategies which build on the prior knowledge of the student
- Repeat for each new situation or activity. PRACTICE, PRACTICE and PRACTICE SOME MORE!

Typical Scenarios where FASD individuals get into trouble

A young FASD adult is on her way home from work with money for bus fare. While waiting for the bus, she spends it on candy and is left with no way to get home.

> *To overcome this problem the person should be issued with a bus pass.*

A young FASD male lends some money to a 'friend' and is surprised that it is not returned- even though they have done this many times before.

> *FASD individuals do not have a good sense of who their 'friends' are. It is best if they do not carry money with them. Or, they should be cued to ask a trusted adult what to do.*

A teenage girl with FASD asks her classmate if she can 'have' her sweater to wear. She is told yes with the unspoken assumption that it is being loaned. The FASD teen will not give the sweater back and argues that it is now hers as her classmate 'gave it to her!

> *The FASD teen does not pick up on the assumed loan of the sweater. She sees it as very black and white and took the literal meaning.*

A FASD child is asked if they have brushed their teeth. The child says that he has, though it is obvious that he has not. The care-giver becomes frustrate by what seems like wilful lying on the child's part.

> *The child is not lying; they probably did brush their teeth at some time. It is important to be specific in asking the questions.*

Chapter 3

Consequences

Many students with FASD are impulsive, saying and doing things we as adults wish they wouldn't. This is an information-gathering problem. The students fail to recognize and evaluate social cues that are presented by those with whom they interact. Unable to sense a classmate's irritation as a result of their behaviour, they are unable to change the offending behaviour until a crisis arises. Subtle cues such as tone of voice, facial expression and body language need to be identified and translated for these students. In addition to these factors, the excitement of the moment often blurs their ability to reflect and think through uncomfortable social situations.

What do we want to accomplish when we discipline? Most adults agree that we want to support children to grow up to be loving and responsible. This must be the measure by which we respond to their wrongdoings. Most of the time the poor social behaviours of the FASD students are more distressing to them than they are to us. This leaves no room for punitive punishment. Research shows that punishment does not work with this population. Power struggles can be avoided by telling students that they may or may not be able to control what they did, but they own their own bodies, so they are responsible for what was said or done.

What works with FASD students is having the students make reparations for wrongdoing as immediately as possible and in the shortest time frame. The hardest thing is for the adult to remain calm and not be reactive. For example, when a student slams the door they can do immediate positive practice- "please go and close the door gently." They can do chores to pay for items they might break or help repair the item. They can come home earlier from an outing next time or stay behind for missed curfew. They can be a helper in the school, thus giving back to the school community and at the same time being able to practice appropriate behaviours. Better still is trying to catch students before they do something wrong and help them think and plan. This is when the most learning takes place. Remember, this is an on-going process and much repetition is needed with each new situation and event. This includes things they have done many times.

When students do make a mistake and get into trouble it is important that they have a way to leave the situation without further embarrassment. Not doing so inevitably ends up in greater misbehaviour. Sometimes the students become so upset and angry they do not recognize that they should leave the room. When this occurs the teacher can use a prearranged signal to cue the student to leave and go to the prearranged quiet and safe spot. This strategy is vital to helping the student hold it together while in school. If behaviour needs to be corrected it is best to do so in private when the student is calm and is able to hear and take in what you are saying. The 'sandwich' technique is useful, praise first, then correction and finish with praise. The goal is to teach accountability by teaching the student how to recognize their signs of over stimulation and build a repertoire of strategies to diffuse blow- ups.

If students are sent to the office to face administrators they must be taught to have an advocate go with them or to ask for their advocate to be there. Due to their poor communication skills they do not perform well under pressure and often end up making the situation worse by swearing or raging. They may also tell the person what they want to hear, by admitting to the deed even if they didn't do it. If there are on-going behavioural issues that cannot be resolved with the advocate role then meetings with the parents/caregivers, support team and educational team are needed to review and discuss medical issues, environmental concerns and other sources of stress.

Special Students Need:

Hope

Possibilities

To build trust

Consistency

Calm in chaos

To build on strengths

Opportunities to shine

Outdoor activities

Patience

Love and acceptance

Carol McAndrew

Chapter 4

Executive Dysfunction

In the brain the frontal lobe conducts the executive functions that are processes involving planning, organization, and other control processes. Most FASD individuals have dysfunction in this lobe. Deficits in executive function seriously challenge the learner. Without the ability to organize and manipulate information an individual with EDF is unable to begin tasks and also complete tasks on their own. Impaired executive function can affect processing speed, which is the rate of work a student can consistently maintain.

Generalizing from one situation to another can also be a problem. FASD individuals are not able to learn easily from their mistakes or successes because they cannot generalize. As a result, what we see is a continuation of the negative behaviour despite negative consequences.

When asked to complete a long-term assignment the FASD student will have difficulty without a "road map" to follow. In an attempt to hide their embarrassment and frustration about the inability to meet the demands of the task the student may appear to be avoiding the assignment.

There is a need for an advocate/mentor to be their "external" brain. This can be something that the FASD individual will balk at, at first. There is a fine line between facilitating success and being perceived as "bossy". Where possible, start with the least intrusive strategy for the individual. Model and discuss the strategy. Start to compile a life skills strategy booklet for each individual with cues and reminders that they can refer to when needed. Creating a checklist for various activities is effective. For example, arrival at school: (If needed have pictures as well)

- Say "good morning" politely

- Take off jacket and hang on the coat peg

- Take agenda out of backpack

- Give agenda to teacher/ teacher assistant

- Hang up back pack on coat peg

- Go directly to your seat

- Sit down quietly and face the front

- Look at the teacher

- Listen for directions for the day

Chapter 5

Communication Skills

FASD individuals have good expressive language skills, but they have poor communication skills. They can appear very sociable and "with it", but they don't always get the right message across and cannot always get the right message from others. Their thoughts get mixed up, they forget and they perceive things differently.

It is important to create a trust relationship with each FASD individual and support and facilitate a process where they automatically ask for help or clarification. The rule of thumb is "always ask for help". For the FASD individual this is when they are not sure; it is the first time they are trying something; they have had problems with this situation in the past; they are confused; they are scared; or a voice in their head says, "I can handle this myself". This is an ongoing life strategy that can help FASD individuals become more self-sufficient.

In our school as in most schools respecting self, others and others' property is valued. It is not enough to just talk about respect, FASD students need to have concrete examples and models of what respect looks like. Here are my guidelines:

What is respect?
- Respect is good manners when you are talking to others, when you are playing, when you are working, when you are at home with your family, when you are at school or work, when you are in public. These can be broken down modelled and practiced. It is helpful to have visual cues too.

- Respect is more than good manners and being polite. It is listening when someone is talking and not interrupting.

- Respect means expressing your anger or frustration without using bad words or name calling or putting people down.

- Respect means giving others their space.

- Respect means keeping your hands and feet to yourself.

- Respect means asking before taking and using other people's things and being able to walk away when the person says no.

- Respect means having a positive attitude with all others.

- Respect means knowing when to take a personal time out.

FASD students must be taught how to communicate their needs and why this is important as a life skill. Modelling and role-playing are effective ways of getting the point across in shaping communication skills. Use everyday examples to create "teachable moments" around expressing needs, feelings and opinions. When needs are verbalized they are more likely to be met. When feelings are discussed, a better understanding between people occurs. Expressing opinions can lead to a better quality of life. The emphasis has to be on that good communication can help prevent problems and arguments.

Here is a scenario from one of my classes. Kay comes into work time for Language Arts. She knows to get her folder and pencil out. She opens her folder and looks at the page of work. She begins to write but within seconds her paper, pencil and folder go flying across the room and she yells, "This is so stupid! I am never doing this again!" Kay could be reprimanded and punished with no recess for her outburst but that is only looking at the outward behaviour. A quick intervention is to remind Kay prior to work time that she can ask for help first when she feels frustrated. "Rewind the scene" is something I use often to have her start again taking Kay through the activity including the positive way to ask for help. She then completes the task successfully and feels good about herself and her abilities. This is not a one shot thing. With each new activity and task the process must be repeated, repeated and repeated some more!!!

Something I do to try to intervene before the outburst, is to be aware that a difficult section is coming up or picking up that it is an unsettled day for Kay and I need to be close by to "jump start" her in the work, removing the stress. I do not ask her if she needs help, rather, I will say, " Wow, this is a tough page, let's start it together. I may need your help on this one." This way too, I can praise Kay for starting and completing the task and review how having my support is helping her learn in a better way. In a class setting it is important to do this technique with all students so the FASD students see that this is a life skill for everyone to learn. This needs to occur with each new task and situation. Setting a student up for success helps lessen their stress and feeling "dumb".

FASD students have a difficult time registering feelings and emotions, so again it is good to help them cue into physical signs. It may be that when they are mad or angry that their faces feel tight and they feel hot. Whatever the triggers, it is good to work to develop warning signs and a repertoire of strategies to help diffuse negative behaviours. Along with trying to tap into the feelings and emotions, it is important to realize that many FASD individuals do not register pain and hurt as normal. I had a high school student who was a distance runner for my high school who ran with a fractured foot!! He did not register the pain fully until it was excruciating. The same goes for self-monitoring for heat and cold. Many days my students would be outside in below zero temperatures without a coat or be bundled up on a plus 30 degree day! They need to be cued as to proper attire. They do not learn from natural consequences like being too cold or too hot.

FASD students love to argue and are quick with putdowns to others. This too is a sign of fear rather than vindictiveness. Having FASD does not excuse rude or hurtful behaviour but the individuals have to learn replacement strategies for negative behaviours. I keep my expectations at school and in the community short and sweet. There is no benefit to justify expectations to FASD students. They operate best where things are black and white. I often phrase things in terms of it is my job to make the "rules" and the students job to follow them. I work towards safety and belonging for all.

We have a "Putdown-free" classroom. Visual reminders are everywhere and reviewed each and every day. Praise and adult attention for positive behaviour is given out. Infractions are dealt with on the spot. Sometimes it is as simple as reminding the students of the "rule" and having them rephrase the putdown into a nicer form of criticism. If the student appears unsettled and rattled then it is best to remove them quietly and take a time out and then discuss the situation in private before having them practice the more polite form of voicing their opinion. Do remember to keep it concise, concrete and pertinent to the immediate situation. Avoid saying such things as, " How many times do I have to tell you that we don't allow put-downs in here!" Stay calm and even in your speaking and model the appropriate way for the student if needed. Sometimes, I do a "rewind of the tape" with all my antics and silliness to get the student out of their funk and have them "do take two" with the "faux pas" dubbed over as they do in the movies. This allows me as the teacher to have the students do the self- correcting right away without me putting them down for what I was calling them to task on.

17

Chapter 6

Building Relationships

Good communication is at the heart of making lasting relationships and friendships. Due to the social impairment of FASD individuals, school personnel and family members often give up on having their students have meaningful relationships. I believe strongly that we can teach relationship development with FASD individuals. Persons with FASD are human beings and I believe that a desire and need for emotion-based relationships is universal to all of the human species. Why do so many FASD individuals in teen years and adulthood suffer from depression and are victims of suicide?

Relationships like any of the academic areas of learning depend upon a foundation of many skills built one upon the other. If the basics of relationships are not mastered, then more complex relationships are very hard to achieve. The skills involved in being a friend differ from social skills. Often in schools we do a good job of teaching social skills as a set of specific behaviours such as making eye contact, taking turns, smiling, hand shakes and asking and answering politely. We role model, script, use social stories and offer practice in the appropriate environments. Somehow though, our FASD students do not seem to learn relationship skills.

Relationship competence requires a careful and systematic layering of skills. I have learned this through the many years of coaching athletes through many levels of track and field. Beginning in a one to one setting with an adult as the coach or facilitator starts the process where there are no distractions and no other demands placed on the individual. The coach is both the guide and participant. The more able partner, the coach, does all the relationship "balancing". Coaching requires careful observation and a different style of communication. As with my track and field coaching I had to find ways to break down the skills for each athlete and work with their personalities, strengths and weaknesses as well as my own!!

It is the same for FASD "athletes". I had to slow down my speech, use fewer words, and amplify and exaggerate my non-verbal communication. As in Track and Field coaching I had to meter my guiding and pacing of new skills and try to stay at the edge of the person's competence for maximum learning potential. Not all goes smoothly, but I have learned from mistakes and worked to modify my approach.

There are several areas that can be developed in building up the scaffolding for relationship building. These include understanding what is meant by friend and acquaintance; providing opportunities to make positive emotional connections with others starting with collaborative play; learning about the give and take in a relationship working towards mutual appreciation and support; managing disagreements and resolving conflicts in a positive manner; handling and coping with disappointment and hurt; creating social memories; accepting people for who they are with their strengths and weaknesses.

Keep in mind when beginning to work on relationship building that each FASD individual comes with different "baggage" and developmental levels of maturity. Many of my students have experienced terrible abuse both physically and mentally. They have been shunted from one foster home to the next with much rejection. They have a great deal of difficulty bonding. Physically they can appear normal but in so many other ways they are delayed in their development. Do not try to rationalize things or lecture to them. The fewer words the better. Actions speak louder than words and that is so true for the FASD individual. Relationship building cannot be foisted upon a person. It needs to be nurtured slowly. There are many programs out there to pull ideas from. Also realize that the term "friend" needs to be clarified from "acquaintance". Many of the students and adults with FASD have taught me this. In an effort to have "friends" they will treat new acquaintances as life-long friends and not be able to distinguish who real friends are. Often, as they move into adolescence and adulthood they migrate to unwise relationships and are taken advantage of.

Having a trusted adult to reference with is needed. This is like the "external brain" providing the missing executive functions. Most FASD adults and young people I have met at conferences and have taught, say that having a parent or care-giver who kept them organized and on track and believing in them is the key to their success.

Another useful strategy to teach about caring and empathy as well as incorporating safety issues, is through bringing in my dog Rocky to the class. FASD students seem to have a natural affinity towards animals. Rocky was a rescued dog from the SPCA in Salmon Arm after being abandoned on the highway and hit by a car. He was in need of love, firmness and consistency in training. He still is not good around vehicles. When he comes into the class the students take turns caring for his physical needs and learn to play with him. He is a great dog for this as he is gentle and very easy-going. The students have learned the difference an "inside" voice makes for Rocky as he is agitated when people speak too loudly. Also, many of my students have issues around road safety so they take turns to "teach" Rocky about stopping and checking for vehicles and crossing carefully on our neighbourhood walks. Although they are training the dog, in reality they are learning themselves!

The FASD students also respond well to hands on learning. Whether guests from the community come in to teach directly or we go to the workplace, is a super way for these students to come alive in their learning. I am in the process of ascertaining some retired members of the community to come in and we will visit them to do crafts together. This is another way to build relationships, especially for the students who are in foster care and do not have extended family close by. Our class is also involved in the many activities offered by the Aboriginal Program. These again are hands on and the students really look forward to them. For the FASD aboriginal students, they are discovering another avenue for building relationships and common cultural backgrounds.

Having the students out of the school building and practicing relationship building and social skills in real life situations works very well. Even within the group, the interactions are much more positive when the pressure of school performance is lessened. We go on a number of field trips, and participate in swimming, bowling and other neat activities such as rock climbing ongoing throughout the year. We study science and social studies and do a great deal of reading and comprehending, problem solving and interpolating through field trip activities.

Through our cooking classes at school, involving some family members, other teachers and teacher assistants, each student has a turn to be the "expert" for the week. International cooking was a big hit with the class. Each student not only chose a country and recipe but collected and shared information with the rest of the class on their chosen ethnic group. They also got to choose a cooking partner so that each class member had a turn as an assistant chef. They were responsible, under adult direction to plan the meal, copy out the recipe, go out and buy the ingredients, research their country, prepare the meal, set the table, serve the food and clean up. It was quite something to see their self-confidence and esteem grow.

Through out the year we took pictures of the many activities the students partook in. These pictures were displayed around the class and in the hallways for others to see. All the students spent some time integrated into regular class activities such as P.E. Fine Arts and Music. We accompanied other classes on field trips. The highlight trip for the students was to the Play Land in Vancouver sponsored by CKNW Orphans Fund.

As a finale to the year, we held a family barbecue at a local nature park. The students had chosen work samples and pictures of activities they were proud of and created a scrapbook for the year. We shared those with parents and celebrated their successes and talents. It was a very emotional time! For many parents/guardians, it was the first time at the end of a school year that they were hearing positive things about their student!! For some, it was a miracle that their student was still in school!!

Chapter 7

Life Skills for Success

It is imperative for FASD students to be exposed over and over again to life skill training. As they don't generalize well from one situation to another, life skills must be taught and repetition is the key. Something as simple as remembering the sorting of laundry will need to be repeated many times for the process to stick. Even for those of us who are not challenged in mind processing, to really learn and retain a skill in long term memory takes 3 weeks. With FASD students and adults it will take a lot more time and if the retrieval system is poor, continuous cues will be needed.

Over the years I have compiled a curriculum to help teach the needed life skills. The students continue to teach me what they need to learn. The curriculum and strategies is constantly being refined as I come to learn what works best. Here is an outline:

Social Skills

Communication Skills	Body Language Cues
	Active listening
Anger Management	Coping Skills –relaxation, self talk
	Asking for help
Friends	Building Relationships
	Circle of Friends
Personal Safety	Picking up on warning signals
Street safety	use of animals to help students cross streets safely

Getting along with co-workers	Who I like to work with
Leisure Skills	Providing choices, card and board Games, recreational sports, clubs

Decision-Making

Providing guidelines	External brain to set up good choices
Money Management	A trusted trustee Shopping skills Record keeping Saving Supervised Spending No bank cards – personal banking skills Creating a budget Paying bills No credit Help with Income tax

Employability Skills

Time Management	Using the external brain to remember
First Day on the Job	Role Play
Proper Dress	Visual cues, personal hygiene issues
Acting Appropriately	Role Play, lists, sequences, key words
Sexual Behaviour	Public versus private behaviour
Quality of the job	What the end product should look like
Safety	Constant review of safety issues
Good Attitude	What this looks like, key words

Using Public Transit

Learning the route	Role Playing and practice with mentor
Cost	Passes are best

Health

Physical Fitness	Mentor to help involve the person in

	life-long fitness and recreation
Nutrition	Daily Food Intake
	Balanced diet
Stress Management	Who do I ask for help
Good Personal Habits	Hygiene, sleep, laundry, cleaning,
	Establishing routines, charts
Medical Issues	Going to the doctor / dentist
Sexuality Training	Understanding the body, birth
	Control (for older students)

Understanding the Law
Where to get help	A mentor/advocate to call

Telephone Skills
Finding phone numbers	Practice with the phone book
Asking for information	Role Play, prompting, script
Work related telephone skills	Role Play, script
How to make long distance calls	Practice, timer

I have had to do a great deal of work with potential employers. Explaining the value of check lists, short directions broken down to one task at a time, concrete language and instructions, checking for understanding, modelling expected outcomes are some of the things I try to develop with the employers. It is important that a familiar face is with the students or adults in starting a new position either in work experience or actual employment. One of my biggest frustrations is that employers often treat the FASD individual as Mentally Challenged and give them mundane tasks to do. This leads to boredom and loss of interest in the job. A girl I knew went to work at a florists and her only task was to cut ends off flowers and put them in water. I think that would drive me a little crazy too. Daily review of expectations is crucial as well as giving the individual tasks they feel valued for.

A caution, many FASD persons feel that once they have learned a skill there is no need to listen to further instructions. Clear delineation of roles is needed and reviewed daily as well as to the quality needed in the end product.

I have seen this too in FASD individuals who go into Special Olympics sports. Once they have mastered how to perform the sport they will argue with the coach and this can set up for major conflict and expulsion from the team. Again, I emphasis the importance of setting out the role of the coach and the athlete very concisely. I use, "this is my job and this is your job".

For the FASD worker, a clear checklist of tasks will help them perform their job more effectively. Cueing for correct social responses is needed daily. For example: a young FASD woman is hired to do nails at a beauty salon. She is very good at performing the needed steps to create a good result. However, she is not good at initiating conversation with the clients or remembering to offer them coffee or other things. Clients see her as rude and forgetful and the boss yells at her yet again for not doing all the social things. She can be forgetful but she only sees the world from her perspective. If she doesn't want a drink of something then why should her client want one? This can be easily rectified with a daily review of expectations and including the social actions into her checklist as well as scripting out some dialogue to get her started. Using humour and redirection is also useful and saves face for her. Unfortunately, too many employers don't want to spend the time to set the FASD person up for success and they are fired.

Chapter 8

Learning the "FASD" Way

Working with a variety of FASD students and adults I have come to appreciate their perspective when it comes to the disabilities they all have in processing and comprehending language. Often many of these students have " wonderful gift of the gab". They appear to be understanding yet in most instances they are lost and have little idea what is expected of them. Some are great word readers but cannot string the words together into a logical understanding. They forget simple steps in processes and do not transfer experiences and learning to new situations. When teachers, parents, care-givers, other professionals and support staff begin to realize this, an "epiphany" can take place!!! Your screams and theirs will be drastically reduced!

Some Simple tips:

Reduce the verbiage. Keep statements simple. " Bob, please sit in your chair" – call them by name then they know you are addressing them.

Give one idea at a time – Allow time for processing of the words. Pay attention to individual signs that they don't get it. Be ready to repeat in a different more concrete way.

Keep a calm and steady tone to your voice.

Tell the person what you want them to do-not what you don't want them to do. "Keep you hands by your sides" rather than, "Don't hit others"

Provide visual cues such as checklists or pictures of a sequence- getting up routine in the morning; the school day class schedule; set up ahead of time any changes that may take place – do with the group and then again with the individual.

Review expectations and routines daily, even from place to place. Do not assume that they remember or transfer from one activity to the next!!!

Continually check for understanding- allow them to respond in their own words; a verbatim regurgitation of words doesn't mean understanding. Watch for signs of non-understanding. Usually each person has some physical sign such as a twitch or such.

Give lots of praise and encouragement that is concrete.
"Thank you for putting your book on the bottom shelf";
"Great job sweeping the crumbs into the dustpan!"
Repeat, repeat, and repeat!!!!

Remember, non-compliance happens for many reasons such as fear, lack of understanding what to do or not knowing how to start.

Chapter 9

The Last Word

It is not rocket science when it comes to supporting FASD individuals. It takes a shift in thinking, flexibility, a great deal of patience and hanging in there for the long haul. As professionals, parents, caregivers and support staff we need to build a sense of team to care for the FASD population as well as work to educate young women and men to the effects of drinking in pregnancy.

There is nothing better than seeing a FASD individual succeed in life, learning to have fun and fulfill their potential. Their smiles and laughter keep me wanting to educate others to their strengths and they continually help me become the person I was meant to be.

I have created a new acronym for FASD:

F   ull of potential

A   dept in special ways

S   eeking acceptance

D   efining resilience

May you find this book useful in helping you on the journey of working with exceptional people, who just happen to have Fetal Alcohol Spectrum Disorder.

Epilogue

I have been a classroom and Special Education teacher for over 25 years. I have experience from Kindergarten to Grade 12 and beyond. Early on, I realized that the main stream of education and its environment did not fit all students. My first year teaching in Castlegar I met a challenging group of junior high students, some of them FASD but undiagnosed, for that was a time when little was known of such a disorder. They taught me what was needed to support their learning and when I put some different strategies into place all the negative behaviours disappeared. I was on my way to a career of working with challenging students.

I do have to say that working with the students that don't fit the system has been so rewarding and has stretched and moulded me as an educator. I have a passion for my job even after such a long time. Days are never boring. I have come to see the world differently and be more flexible in all I do. FASD students have taught me so much as well as the families I have had the pleasure to work with. I continue to meet new people and make new connections.

Seeing youngsters come alive and shine in so many areas of expertise is so uplifting for me. Some of these are in music, singing, drumming and dance, basketball, track and field and Special Olympics for skiing, track and baseball. Some have taught me patience in learning to bead and also a window into the aboriginal culture. I do become emotionally attached and I think that is the key to building up a trust relationship. So many of these individuals have had such heartache and hurt in their lives they do not bond easily. I think of their trust in me as a great privilege and it is so rewarding to see them smile, honestly laugh, be relaxed and enjoy themselves.

Presently, I am teaching in Langley in a unique multi-grade district program that has developed to accommodate multi-needs of students with FASD, Asperger's Syndrome, Tourette's Syndrome, OCD (Obsessive

29

Compulsive Disorder), ADHD (Attention Deficit Disorder) and combinations of these. It is a challenging job but one I love. I work with three incredible teacher assistants and together we team to meet the needs of the students. For most of the participants, it is the first time that they have been able to attend school full time and for the entire year.

Being a part of FASD Initiative groups in the Okanagan and Shuswap regions as well as presenting workshops throughout B.C. to local and international audiences helps me to grow in my knowledge of FASD and I meet some incredible people along the way.

My hope is that FASD will be properly recognized and more education be done in prevention as this is a totally preventable disorder. For those who have FASD may books like mine help others to have a better understanding of the disorder and work to support all FASD individuals become who they were meant to be.

Resources

Web site links
www.come-over.to/FAS

www3.sk.sympatico.ca/skfasnet
e-mail fas.esupportnetwork@sasktel.net

FASSY (Fetal Alcohol Syndrome Society Yukon)
fascap@yknet.ca

www.fasbookshelf.com

www.fasalaska.com

www.depts.washington.edu/fasdpn

www.acbr.com/fas FASLINK

www.fasworld.com
www.hss.state.ak.us/fas

www.dotolearn.com

Other Helpful Resources
Fantastic Antone Succeeds (1993) and Fantastic Antone Grows Up (2000)
Kleinfield, J
University of Alaska Press, These books give positive experiences of parents,

educators, therapists and researchers with children, adolescents and adults with FASD. They give hope and intervention ideas..

Trying Differently Rather Than Harder
Malbin, D. (2001)
This booklet is written to provide useful information, increase understanding of FAS, reduce frustration, and develop appropriate intervention and prevention strategies.
Order through www.fascets.org

The Best I Can Be
Kulp, L. (2003)
This is written by a FASD teen

Our FAScinating Journey
Kulp, J. (2003)
A family's retelling of living and coping with FASD

Relationship Development Intervention with Children, Adolescents and Adults.
Gutstein, S.E. and Sheely, R. (2002)
Order through the Canadian ASD Centre, Edmonton.

The Explosive Child
Greene, R.W. Dr.
Great strategies for learning to handle easily frustrated and hard to manage children.

Appendix

Figure 1 Behaviour/Function Mapping- A story about our student

TO BE COMPLETED BY THE CLASSROOM TEACHER/OTHER SUPPORT STAFF BEFORE PLANNING/SCHOOL-BASED TEAM MEETINGS AND/OR BY THE SCHOOL- BASED TEAM/FOCUS TEAM.

Student Strengths

I have a student in my class named _____. He/she is in Grade ____. His/her strengths are (Choose from list or add your own) art, music, computers, sports, interacting with/helping others, humour, creativity, leadership, certain academics, entertaining, problem-solving.

Problem Behaviour

When this student struggles or acts out it typically looks like this: (Choose from the list) work refusal, tattling, yelling out, constant inattention, easily distracted, defiance, non-compliance, inappropriate verbalizations, being unprepared, poor attendance, tardy, disruptive, withdrawn, anxious, and/or power struggles.

Precipitating Factors

He/she seems to struggle or act out during: (Choose from list) unstructured

33

times, difficult tasks, particular academics, seat-work, new situations, transitions, small group settings, being around certain individuals, onerous tasks, changes in routines, changes in staff, peer provocation, social isolation, and/or after certain directives, requests made of them.

Triggering Antecedent

Look for patterns- time, duration, subject area, particular individuals. This typically occurs just *before* the behaviour.

Contributing Factors/Setting Events

It is always worse for this child when he/she: (Choose from list) has negative interactions/conflicts with adults/peers (history of peer conflicts), has a difficult start to the morning, missed meals, lack of sleep, conflict at home, has a difficult bus ride/ walk to school, has academic difficulties (history of failure), past school suspension, or expulsion, and/or misses medication.

Negative Reinforcers

Looking at the adult response to the problem behaviour, what generally occurs for the student is: (Choose from list) sent from the classroom, sent to the office, detention, suspension (in-school, out of school), negative adult attention. This is typically what occurs *following* the problem behaviour.

Hypothesis of Function of Behaviour

I think this student might be using this behaviour to: (Choose from list or add your own) obtain teacher/peer attention, obtain a desired objective or activity, escape an undesirable activity, demand/and or people, escape sensory input, escape setting, maintain control, self preservation

---

Desired Behaviours

I wish the child would: (Choose from list) complete the tasks, cooperate with

me/others, come prepared to class, show respect for self/others, use positive self-management strategies, and/or be able to stop/start activities on their own.

Positive Reinforcers

If the student could engage in this positive/desired behaviour, it would likely be maintained because he/she would (Choose from list) have strategies to work through difficult situation, receive positive attention/affirmations from me/peers/ others, build skills/confidence, receive positive feedback on work, and/or feel good about their accomplishments.

Alternative/Replacement Strategies

Since it will take some time for the student to learn and adopt new behaviour practices, in the meantime, I am willing to accept that the student will use approximate behaviours until they reach the desired behaviour such as (choose from list) ask for help in a polite way, ask to work in a different setting, ask politely to take a break, politely decline, and/or propose choices, restore sense of justice.

What is the Function of the Behaviour?
Developing a Hypothesis
Function Mapping (figure 2)

Contributing Factors	Precipitating Factors	
Problem Behaviour	Reinforcers	FUNCTION
	(Negative)	

Behaviour Mapping- Objectives and Strategies
(Figure 3)

Student Strengths   Strategies   Contributing
Precipitating   Behaviour   Reinforcement
                                 Already Tried   Event Strategies Event
Strategies   Teaching Strategies   Strategies

Function Mapping-Building Competing Pathways
(Figure 4)

Desired Behaviours   **Reinforcers (positive)**

Contributing Factors   Precipitating Factors
Problem Behaviour   Reinforcers   Function
                              (negative)

Alternative Replacement Behaviours
Reinforcers (positive)

Acknowledgments

I would like to thank the personnel of School District #35, Langley, B.C. for sharing the Functional Assessment Process with me. I am grateful to my husband, Bruce, who helped me through some of the technical things to do with the computer. A big thank you also goes out to my Mum, Ellen, who was a great editor. Most of all, I thank the young people I have had the privilege to teach and learn so much from in understanding FASD.